Fitness Dice

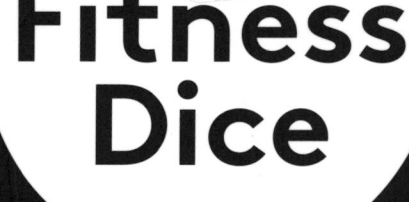

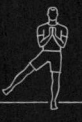

Copyright © 2020 by Chronicle Books LLC.

All rights reserved. No part of this book may be reproduced in any form without written permission from the publisher.

ISBN: 978-1-4521-8238-4

Manufactured in China.

Design by Rachel Harrell.
Text by Jennie Votel, NASM certified personal trainer.
Ilustrations by Arthur Mount.

If you experience discomfort, pain, or extreme breathlessness, stop exercising immediately.

The information, techniques, and exercises presented in this book should not be construed as medical advice and are not meant to replace treatment by licensed health professionals. Please consult your doctor or professional healthcare advisor to determine your body's needs and limitations. The writer and publisher hereby disclaim any liability from injuries resulting from following any recommendation in this book.

10 9 8 7 6 5

Chronicle Books LLC
680 Second Street
San Francisco, CA 94107
www.chroniclebooks.com

CONGRATULATIONS ON YOUR CHOICE TO GET AND STAY FIT!

With thousands of possible combinations, these dice offer a fun and easy way to add variety to your workout routine—at home or on the go.

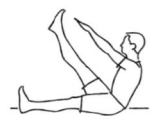

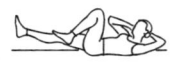

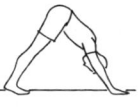

CONTENTS

This kit includes 7 dice and an instructional booklet. There are 6 exercise dice, each focusing on a different area of the body or type of exercise:

- Lower Body
- Upper Body
- Chest and Back
- Core
- Cardio
- Full Body

The seventh die indicates the amount of repetitions (10, 12, 15, or 20) or time (30 seconds or 1 minute) for each exercise.

HOW TO USE THE DICE

Simply roll the 7 dice, then match the numbered illustrations on the dice to the corresponding exercises in the booklet, where you'll find instructions on how to complete each exercise. Perform each exercise for the amount of reps or time rolled.

Please note: These are suggestions. Feel free to do the number of reps you want! Listen to your body and do what feels right.

The workouts can be as long or short as you like, depending on the number of dice you roll and how many times you roll them. If you choose to roll the dice multiple times, do the set of exercises, recover for 1 minute, then roll again. Aim to complete these workouts 3 to 4 times a week.

SUGGESTED ROUTINES

Routine 1: Full Body (all 7 dice)

Routine 2: Upper Body and Cardio

Routine 3: Lower Body and Core

TIPS

Before beginning any workout, it's important to do a warm-up—a walk or jog around the block or a few trips up and down any nearby stairs. After you warm up, you can also do some quick stretches, holding each stretch for 15 seconds.

While performing these exercises, focus on good form (to minimize injury) and controlling your breath (exhaling on the more difficult part of each exercise). If you are just beginning to work out, take it slow. If the exercises are too difficult in the beginning, look for the "make it easier" options within the booklet. If it feels like too much, do fewer reps or take a break. When you are ready to take it up a notch, add on the "extra challenge" options.

Once you've completed your workout, take some time to cool down with light walking and longer stretches, holding each stretch for 30 seconds or more.

Now let's get this workout rolling!

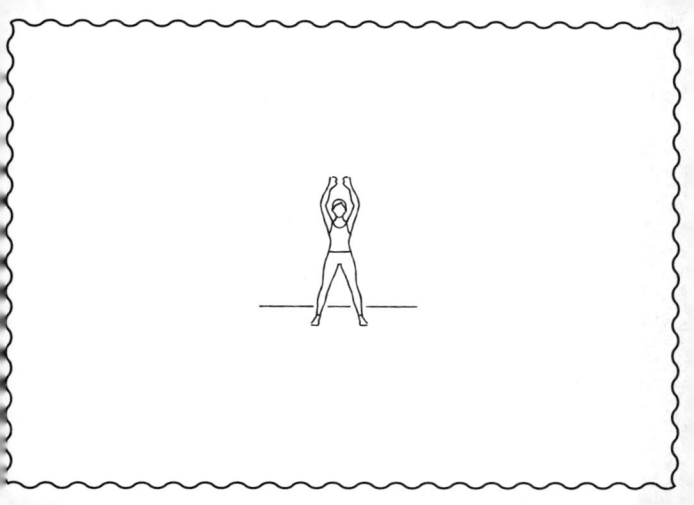

LOWER BODY

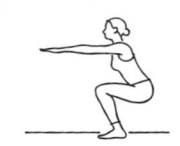

1

SQUATS

Start standing, feet slightly wider than hip-width apart, arms extended forward at shoulder height, palms facing down. Press your heels into the ground as you lower your hips toward the back of your heels. Keep your knees behind your toes, chest lifted, and shoulder blades strong; don't round your back. Press through your heels, squeeze your glutes, and return to start. Repeat this movement for the amount of reps or time rolled. **Make it easier:** Only lower hips to knee level. **Extra challenge:** Squat jumps—from squat position, jump straight up, raising your arms above your head, then return to squat.

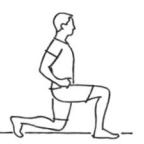

LUNGES

Start standing, feet hip-width apart, hands on hips. Step forward with your right foot, bending the right knee until the top of your leg is parallel to the ground, keeping your knee above your heel. Bend your back leg so your left knee moves toward the ground. Keep your chest up with your spine tall. Press your right heel into the floor and step back to start. Repeat movement with your left foot stepping forward. That's one rep; continue for the amount of reps or time rolled. **Extra challenge:** When lunging, sweep both arms overhead, palms facing in.

3

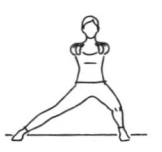

LOWER BODY

LATERAL LUNGES

Start standing, feet hip-width apart, arms by your sides. Take a long step out to the side with your right foot, bending your right knee, sitting back into your hip, and keeping your left leg straight. As you step, extend your arms forward at shoulder height, palms facing in. Keep your right knee above your right heel, with both feet pointed forward. Press into your right heel, squeeze your glute, and return to start, lowering your arms. Repeat on your left side. That's one rep; continue for the amount of reps or time rolled. **Extra challenge:** Add a hop between lunges, reaching both arms above your head.

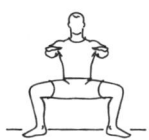

SUMO SQUATS

Start standing, feet much wider than hip-width apart, toes pointing out slightly, arms by your sides. With a straight back, bend your knees until your legs are parallel to the ground. As you lower into a squat, extend your arms forward at shoulder height, palms facing down. Pause, press your weight into your heels, then return to start. Repeat this movement for the amount of reps or time rolled. **Extra challenge:** Start with arms reaching overhead. As you squat, pull your arms down, bringing your elbows to your ribcage. As you stand, reach arms up.

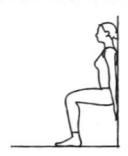

WALL SITS

Stand with your back flat against a wall, walk your feet forward, and lower your hips into a chair position, forming a 90° angle at your knees and hips. Press into your heels, arms by your sides. Hold the position for 5 seconds, then slide back up. That's one rep; continue for the number of reps rolled or hold a static wall sit for the amount of time rolled. **Extra challenge:** Clasp your hands together behind your head with your elbows wide.

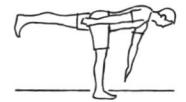

SINGLE-LEG TOUCHDOWNS

Start standing, feet hip-width apart, arms by your sides. Shift your weight onto your right leg and lean forward at the hip as you lift your left leg off the ground behind you, foot flexed. While leaning forward, reach your left hand toward your right toes. Keep your back straight. Press into your right heel and return to start. Repeat for half the amount of reps or time rolled, then switch sides.
Extra challenge: As you lean forward, touch your toe or the ground.

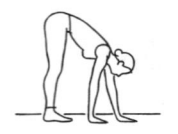

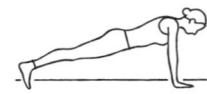

INCHWORMS

Stand with feet hip-width apart. Bend at the waist with legs straight, and place your hands on the floor. Slowly walk your hands forward until they are under your shoulders and you are in a plank position. Pause, then, with legs straight, take small steps forward until your feet are as close to your hands as they can get. Repeat this movement for the amount of reps or time rolled. **Make it easier:** Take a wider stance. **Extra challenge:** Add a push-up when you reach plank position.

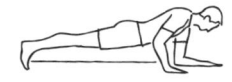

UP-DOWN PLANKS

Hold a forearm plank position with your elbows directly under your shoulders, legs extended. With little to no movement in the hips, press your right palm into the floor followed by your left palm, straightening your arms. Pause, then return your right forearm to the floor, followed by your left forearm. Repeat this movement for half the amount of reps or time rolled, then switch, leading with the left side: left hand, right hand, left forearm, right forearm. **Make it easier:** Drop to your knees with your feet in the air.

UPPER BODY 9

TRICEPS DIPS

Sit with knees bent, feet flat on the floor, hip-width apart. Place your palms behind you, directly under your shoulders, fingers pointing toward your body. Lift your hips off the ground, straightening your arms. Shift your weight back onto your hands, opening your chest. Bend your elbows to lower yourself down. That's one rep; continue for the amount of reps or time rolled. **Extra challenge:** Lift one leg parallel to the floor while completing the exercise. Repeat for half the amount of reps or time rolled, then switch sides.

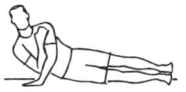

SIDE-LYING TRICEPS PUSH-UPS

Start lying on your right side with legs extended and stacked. Wrap your right arm around your chest and hold your left shoulder with your right hand. Place your left hand on the ground in front of your chest. Press your left hand into the floor, engage your triceps, and straighten your arm, lifting your upper body off the floor. Pause at the top, then return to start. Repeat for half the amount of reps or time rolled, then switch sides. **Extra Challenge:** Keep your knees bent and tucked behind you.

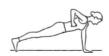

PUSH-UP TO ROW

Start in plank position, hands under your shoulders, arms straight, legs extended. Bend your elbows and lower your chest toward the ground into a push-up, then press back up and pull your right arm up toward the right side of your ribcage, with your elbow coming up behind your shoulder blade. Pause, then return to start. Repeat on the left side. That's one rep; continue for the amount of reps or time rolled. **Make it easier:** Keep your knees on the ground with your feet in the air.

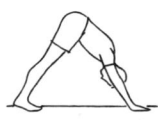

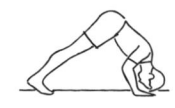

PIKE PUSH-UPS

Start in plank position, hands under your shoulders, arms straight, legs extended. Lift your hips high so your legs and chest form an inverted-V shape (pike position). Leading with your forehead, bend your elbows and bring your head toward the floor. Pause before you touch the ground and press back to pike. Repeat this movement for the amount of reps or time rolled. **Make it easier:** Do it on your knees. **Extra challenge:** Stand on your tiptoes in pike position before lowering your head toward the ground.

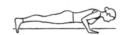

PUSH-UPS

Start in plank position, hands slightly wider than your shoulders, arms straight, legs extended. Keeping your core engaged, bend your elbows and lower your chest toward the ground. Pause at the lowest point, right before you touch the ground, then return to start. Repeat this movement for the amount of reps or time rolled. **Make it easier:** Drop to your knees with feet in the air or position your hands on a sofa, low step, or countertop, rather than the floor. **Extra challenge:** Single-leg push-ups—complete the exercise with one leg lifted. Repeat for half the amount of reps or time rolled, then switch sides.

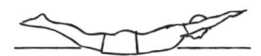

SUPERMANS

Start lying face down, arms outstretched above your head, palms facing down, legs extended. Exhale as you press your hips into the floor and lift your arms, shoulders, and legs 2 to 4 in [5 to 10 cm] off the ground. Gaze down, keeping your neck in line with your spine. Pause, then return to start. Repeat this movement for the amount of reps or time rolled. **Make it easier:** Only lift your chest and arms off the floor; keep feet and legs grounded.

CHEST & BACK

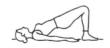

BRIDGES

Start lying faceup with knees bent, feet on the floor, hip-width apart. Keep your hands by your hips, palms facing down. As you exhale, press your feet and shoulders into the floor and lift your hips off the ground as high as you can. Pause at the top, then return to start. Repeat this movement for the amount of reps or time rolled. **Extra challenge:** Extend your left leg off the ground and perform the bridge with only your right foot. Repeat for half the amount of reps or time rolled, then switch sides.

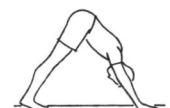

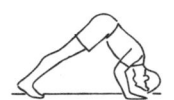

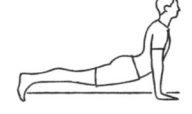

DIVE BOMBER PUSH-UPS

Start in plank position, hands slightly wider than your shoulders, arms straight, legs extended. Lift your hips high so your legs and chest form an inverted-V shape (pike position). As your bend your elbows into a push-up, lower your chest toward the ground between your hands. As you drive your chest through your hands, lift your head and chest toward the sky, pressing through your hands and straightening your arms. Return to pike and repeat for the amount of reps or time rolled. **Make it easier:** Do the exercise on your knees with feet in the air.

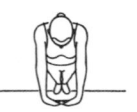

TRICEPS PUSH-UPS

Start in plank position, hands in a diamond shape under the center of your chest, arms straight, legs extended. Bend your elbows and lower your chest toward the floor, squeezing your elbows in tight toward your ribcage as you lower down. Pause at the lowest point, right before you touch the ground, then return to start, keeping your elbows close to your torso throughout the exercise. Continue for the amount of reps or time rolled. **Make it easier:** Drop to your knees with feet in the air or use a sofa, low step, or countertop for your hands, rather than the floor.

I/Y/T

Start lying face down, arms outstretched above your head, palms facing down, legs extended. Exhale as you press your hips into the floor, lifting your arms off the ground, forming the letter "I." Squeeze your legs together as you lift. Pause, then return to start. Repeat the lift with hands slightly wider, forming the letter "Y." Pause and lower. Repeat the lift with hands straight out to the side, forming the letter "T." That's one rep; continue cycling through I/Y/T for the amount of reps or time rolled. **Extra challenge:** Lift your legs off the floor as you lift your arms.

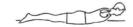

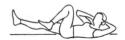

BICYCLE CRUNCHES

Lie faceup, hands behind head, elbows wide. Bring your knees to a 90° angle with feet off the floor. Keeping your lower back on the floor, lift your shoulder blades and bring your right elbow toward your left knee while extending your right leg. Pause, then switch. That's one rep; continue for the amount of reps or time rolled. If your back is coming off the floor, keep your knees slightly bent and reach your heels toward the floor. **Make it easier:** Keep one foot on the floor and bring your opposite knee in toward your chest.

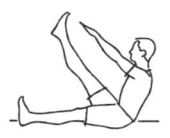

V-UPS

Start lying faceup, arms reaching overhead, touching the ground, legs extended. As you exhale, sit up and reach your hands toward your toes while lifting your right leg up, creating a V shape with your upper body and right leg. Slowly roll back down to start and repeat with your left leg. That's one rep; continue for the amount of reps or time rolled. **Make it easier:** Only lift your shoulders off the floor, rather than fully sitting up. **Extra challenge:** Lift both feet up, rather than alternating legs.

TWIST WITH A LIFT

Sit with knees bent, heels on the floor, hip-width apart. Keeping your chest lifted, lean back until your abs engage. Clasp your hands together and extend your arms in front of your chest, keeping your back straight. Sweep your hands back behind your right hip, pause, then sweep your hands up above your head, sitting up tall. Immediately bring your hands to your left hip as you lean back slightly. Pause, then sweep your hands back overhead as you sit up. That's one rep; continue for the amount of reps or time rolled.

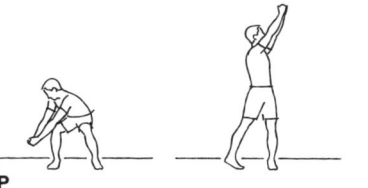

CROSS CHOP

Stand tall with feet slightly wider than hip-width apart. Squat slightly with knees over your heels, clasp your hands together, and reach toward the outside of your right knee, twisting at the waist. Pause and swing your clasped hands away from your body and up toward your left shoulder while twisting your torso and pivoting on your right foot. At the top of the exercise, your arms should be straight, with your upper arms in front of your face. Return to a squat and repeat for half the amount of reps or time rolled, then switch sides.

PLANK JACKS

Start in plank position, hands under your shoulders, arms straight, legs extended. Jump your feet out to the side, pause, and jump back to start. Be sure to squeeze your glutes, with little movement through the hips. Your belly button should be pulled toward your spine to stabilize your core as you repeat this movement for the amount of reps or time rolled. **Make it easier:** Tap your left foot out to the left and back to center; repeat with your right foot.

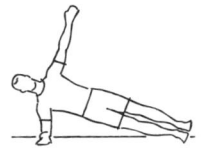

SIDE-PLANK TAPS

Lie on your right side with legs extended and stacked, right forearm directly under shoulder, palm on the floor. Pressing your forearm into the floor, lift your knees and hips up, reaching your left arm into the air with your palm facing forward. Hold this position as you dip your right hip toward the floor, then lift back up. Continue dipping for half the amount of reps or time rolled, then switch sides. **Make it easier:** Bend both knees with feet stacked or let your bottom knee rest on the floor and extend the top leg.

24

CORE

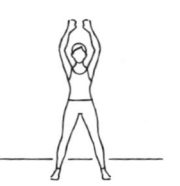

JUMPING JACKS

Start standing, feet together, arms by your sides. Jump your feet out to the side while bringing your arms together above your head. Jump back to start. Continue for the amount of reps or time rolled. **Make it easier:** Take out the jump and tap one foot out to the side as you raise your arms; repeat with the opposite foot. **Extra challenge:** Squat jack—as you jump into your wide stance, lower your hips and reach your hands toward the ground, pause, and jump back to start. Keep your back straight.

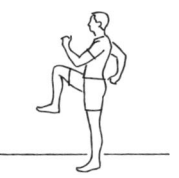

HIGH KNEES

Start standing, feet together, arms by your sides. Lift your right knee quickly up to hip height as you bend your left elbow and bring your left hand toward your left shoulder. Quickly return to start and repeat on the opposite side, running in place. That's one rep; continue for the amount of reps or time rolled. **Make it easier:** March in place rather than running. Try to get knees to hip height while moving your arms quickly.

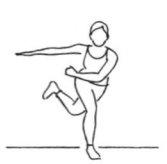

SPEED SKATERS

Stand with feet together, arms by your sides. Shift your weight onto your left foot and hop to the right as if jumping over a mat, landing on your right foot with your knee slightly bent, swinging your left knee behind your right knee, and keeping your left foot off the ground. Allow your arms to swing across the front of your body as you hop. Pause, and repeat on the left. That's one rep; continue for the amount of reps or time rolled. **Make it easier:** Step from side to side rather than jumping.

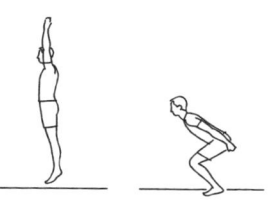

SKIER HOPS

Stand with feet together, arms by your sides. Reach both arms above your head and jump with both feet to the right, keeping your knees together. As you land, push your arms straight back behind your hips, pausing in a squat, then lift your arms back above your head and jump to the left side. As you land, lower your arms straight back, pausing in a squat. That's one rep; continue jumping from side to side for the amount of reps or time rolled. **Make it easier:** Step your feet from side to side.

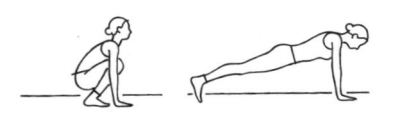

BURPEES

Stand with feet hip-width apart, arms by your sides. Bend your knees and place your hands on the ground, shoulder-width apart. Jump or step your feet back so you are in a plank position. Bend your elbows and lower your chest toward the floor in a push-up. Straighten your arms back to a plank. Jump or step your feet in toward your hands and stand up. That's one rep; continue for the amount of reps or time rolled. **Make it easier:** Take out the push-up. **Extra challenge:** Add a jump between reps.

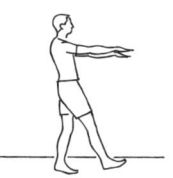

MUMMY KICKS

Stand with feet hip-width apart, arms extended forward at shoulder height, palms facing down. Keeping your core engaged and your arms and legs straight, kick your right foot out in front of you while crossing your right arm over your left. Then kick your left foot forward, crossing your left arm over your right. That's one rep; continue alternating at a fast pace for the amount of reps or time rolled.

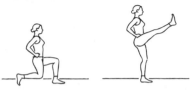

REVERSE LUNGE WITH FRONT KICK

Stand with feet hip-width apart, hands on hips. Step back with your right foot into a lunge, bending your left knee at a 90° angle, with your left knee above your left heel and weight in your left foot. Pause in the lowest position, with your right knee almost touching the floor. Drive your right foot forward into a front kick, then immediately step back with your right foot and repeat. Continue for half the amount of reps or time rolled, then switch sides. **Make it easier:** Skip the kick and simply drive your knee up to hip height.

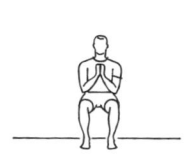

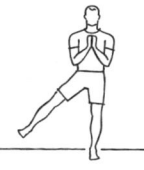

SQUAT WITH SIDE LEG LIFT

Start standing, feet hip-width apart, hands clasped in front of your chest. Bend your knees and lower your hips back into a squat. Keep your weight in your heels and pause in the lowest position. Drive up through your heels, coming out of the squat and lifting your right leg straight out to the side with your foot flexed. Place your foot back on the ground and return to start. Repeat the squat and, as you rise up, lift your left leg to the side. That's one rep; continue for the amount of reps or time rolled.

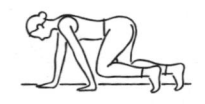

BEAR CRAWL

Start on all fours, hands under your shoulders, knees directly below hips. Engage your core and lift your knees so they are hovering just above the floor. Keeping your back flat and hips steady, move your right hand and left foot forward. Pause briefly, then move your left hand and right foot forward, keeping your knees off the floor. Take three steps forward with each hand and foot, then move backward to return to start. That's one rep; continue for the amount of reps or time rolled.

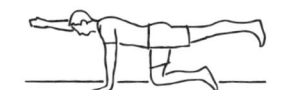

BIRD DOG

Start on all fours, hands under your shoulders, knees directly below hips. Engage your core and keep your back straight. Extend your right arm straight out at shoulder level, palm facing in, as you extend your left leg straight behind you, foot flexed, toes toward the ground. The leg should be parallel to the floor. Pause, then return to start. Repeat with the left arm and right leg. That's one rep; continue for the amount of reps or time rolled.

FULL BODY

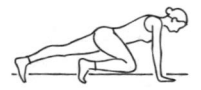

MOUNTAIN CLIMBERS

Start in plank position, hands under your shoulders, arms straight, legs extended. Keeping your back straight and abs engaged, lift your right foot off the floor and tuck your right knee up toward your chest. Pause, then return to start. Repeat with your left knee. That's one rep; continue for the amount of reps or time rolled. **Extra challenge:** Pick up the pace, as if running in plank; be sure to keep your hips low, and do not allow your lower back to sink or your hips to rise.

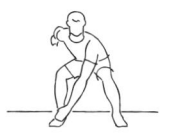

SIDE-SHUFFLE TAPS

Stand with feet hip-width apart, arms by your sides. Squat slightly with hips reaching backward and take two quick side shuffles to the right, making sure both toes stay pointed forward. Reach your left hand down toward the floor to touch your right toes. Then quickly shuffle three steps to the left. Reach your right hand down to touch your left toes. That's one rep; continue for the amount of reps or time rolled. **Make it easier:** Reach toward your knees instead of your toes.

CHRONICLE BOOKS
SAN FRANCISCO

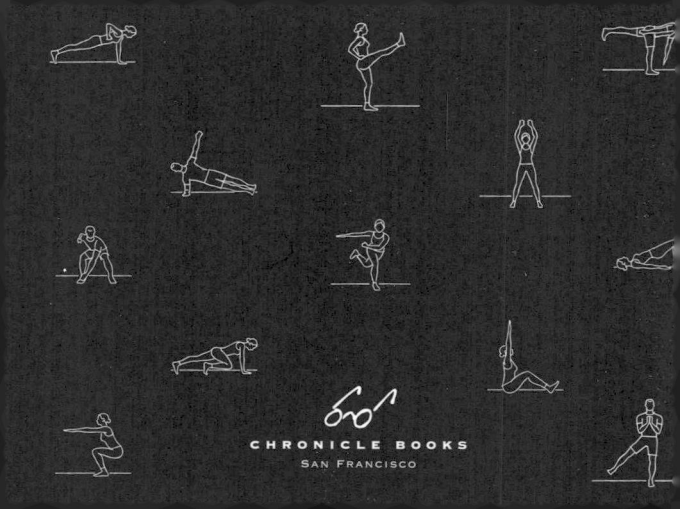